BASIC AB WORKOUTS
GIVE YOU SEXY FLAT ABS

Your One Stop Flat Abs Resource

Ab Exercises Series

Michael Weston

Table of Contents

BASIC AB WORKOUTS GIVE YOU SEXY FLAT ABS

Your One Stop Flat Abs Resource

Ab Exercises Series

"Tried and True Basic Ab Workouts Give You Sexy Flat Abs That Look Great. . .

On the Beach - At the Pool - In the Bedroom!"

My name is Michael Weston. I'm not a fitness guru though I do offer quite a number of specific workouts to help you get those flat abs you've been dreaming about. My background is in clinical psychology (I earned my master's degree quite a few years ago) and nutrition (college level training here, too).

There are three areas you need to focus on when trying to change to way you look: physical exercises, proper nutrition, and how you think about what you're trying to do.

Using proper technique while exercising and eating the right amounts and kinds of foods are important, but let's face it . . . you can learn most of the things you need to know about technique and nutrition from any good physical fitness program.

I enjoy helping others get started on their amazing journey of self-improvement. And I'd like to help you, too. The *Basic Ab Workouts* book contains excellent information about how to get those sexy flat abs you've been dreaming about. You'll also learn:

- **Why it's important when trying to change the way you look to work on all 3 areas -- exercise technique, nutrition, conditioning your mind for success -- simultaneously to get the most benefit out of your efforts**
- Having a large, protruding midsection has far more serious implications than just an unattractive appearance. Find out which life threatening disease becomes much more of a "risk factor" if your tummy gets to where you want to go before the rest of you . . . and what to do to avoid it
- **How to determine whether now is really the right time for you to be trying to change your appearance. Are your reasons for beginning this journey yours or somebody else's? Does it make any difference?**
- Useful information about the names and locations of the abdominal muscle group that could keep you from falling prey to unproven exercise claims as well as keep you from injuring yourself while performing your exercises
- **Proper nutrition is just as important as proper exercise technique when attempting to flatten that tummy and see those abs! We'll examine protein, carbohydrate and fat and see how they contribute to your overall health -- or lack of same**
- I'll tell you an easy way to cut down on your caffeine and sugar intake so you'll be more relaxed and less susceptible to energy highs and lows. (No, not by giving up coffee!)

- **How you think about what you're trying to accomplish has a definite impact on its outcome. But all the positive thinking in the world won't get you where you want to go -- unless you do this, too!**
- Much, much more!

Basic Ab Workouts Give You Sexy Flat Abs

Essential Ab Workouts Information Worth Knowing

Want sexy, ripped flat abs? Many people do. Well, ab workouts are the way to get there.

Most people just want to show off their bare midriffs and feel confident about how good they look, but achieving great abs goes beyond just looks. There are many side benefits of tightening and strengthening your abdominal muscles. For example, a major function of abdominal muscles is to protect and support your viscera (internal abdominal organs). They do this best and most effectively when they are well toned. Weak abs allow the abdomen to become pendulous resulting in a "potbelly."

Your abdominal muscles also support your trunk and have a market effect on posture and movement. They also assist in helping you breathe. Other benefits of well-toned abs include improved core strength, which improves your back alignment and helps to reduce back and neck strain, and helps with just feeling better overall.

It's important that your ab exercises target all of your ab muscles. They are pairs of muscles on either side of your body and consist of:

1) Rectus Abdominus — A medial superficial muscle pair extending from the pubis to the rib cage; ensheathed by aponeuroses (attachments) of lateral muscles; segmented by 3 tendinous intersections. Actions:
– flex and rotate lumbar region of vertebral column
– fix and depress ribs
– stabilize pelvis during walking
– increase intra-abdominal pressure

2) External Oblique — Largest and most superficial of the 3 lateral muscles; fibers run downward and medially (same direction out-stretched fingers take when hands put into pants pockets); aponeurosis turns under inferiorly, forming inguinal ligament. Actions:
– When pair contracts simultaneously, aid rectus abdominus muscles in flexing vertebral column and in compressing abdominal wall and increasing abdominal pressure

– acting individually, aid muscles of back to trunk rotation and lateral flexion

3) Internal Oblique — Most fibers run upward and medially, however the muscle fans so its interior fibers run downward and medially. Actions:
– same as external oblique

4) Transverse Abdominus — Deepest (innermost) muscles of the abdominal wall; fibers run horizontally. Actions:
– compresses abdominal contents

Although you can't touch the transverse abdominus, they have a tremendous effect on posture. Since the fibers run horizontally, they wrap around the body and have a similar effect to wearing a back support belt.

The results from ab workout exercises vary from person to person, some seeing results quickly; others struggling. The reasons for this also vary. It might be that they are targeting the muscles differently. Or, perhaps they're not intensifying their workout as they progress with it over time. Or, maybe they're just doing the wrong exercises altogether. Though any exercise can be an ab exercise, it only becomes one if you tighten your abs while doing it. For example, to use cardio and other exercises as ab exercises, tighten your abs as if you were going to get punched in the stomach while doing them.

Getting the abs of your dreams will definitely give you a boost in confidence. More than that, though, getting the abs of your dreams will also improve your overall health, strength, posture and dexterity.

Reference:

Marieb, Elaine N. Human Anatomy and Physiology, 5th edition. Pearson Education, Inc. c. 2001. p. 346.

BodyBuilding Ab Workouts Give You Sexy Flat Abs

Professional body builders flaunt themselves in TV ads devised to sell you pills, powders, diet supplements, or workouts. However, not everyone thinks a muscle-bound hulk looks attractive or aspires to look like one. This article is not about getting 6-pack abs. It's about flattening your tummy and getting sexy flat abs.

Surely, everyone would like to know the secret of getting slim and maintaining it forever. Well, the secret is that you get nothing, if you invest nothing. In this article, I tell you what you need to do, to look sexy and attractive.

I run you through some bodybuilding ab workouts that can help you. I also tell you about some precautions you need to take, if you want to keep injury at bay while you attain your goal.

My list of best bodybuilding ab workouts includes upper body lifts done keeping your legs straight or bent at the knee, exercise ball workouts, crunches done while hanging from supports, upper body lift crunches done hanging upside down, bench supported crunches done on an inclined bench, crunches done simultaneously with weight training, cycling crunches done lying on the floor, and reverse crunches done by lifting your legs, instead of your upper body.

These bodybuilding ab workouts are a set of exercises that work on each of the muscles in the abdomen (or core, as it is known among gym goers). These muscles are the Rectus Abdominis (the longest and mostly noticed), the External and Internal abdominal Obliques, the Transverse Abdominis and the Pectoralis Major.

Most Effective Crunches

Among the most effective bodybuilding ab workouts are crunches done on the floor either keeping your legs straight or folded. Lie flat back on the floor, bend your legs at the knee such as to form inverted V's, and pull your upper body up till you can touch your knee with your chin. You can ask someone to hold your toes, for added stability. Keep your knees together all the time. Repeat this ten times. Once you reach the top position, hold for four to five seconds, and then slowly lay back down. Repeat the set four times, with intervals of 30 to 40 seconds, between sets.

You can do these with your arms behind your head, crossed over your chest, or holding a weight on your chest. This exercise can also be done over an inclined bench for additional angles and difficulty levels.

Captains Chair Crunches

You could do another form of crunches, using what's called the Captains Chair. If you have well developed leg muscles, they would act as weights. Support yourself in the chair, bring your legs together and lift your legs till they are level with your hips. Repeat ten times. Repeat this set 40 to 50 times, with intervals of rest in between. This is a very good exercise for your lower abs.

When You Feel Like Stopping – Just Stop

Your enthusiasm for workouts could easily lead you to go overboard on exercise routines. Never overdo workouts. After repeating a set, if you feel like stopping, just stop. When you overdo muscle building exercises, you actually end up damaging muscles instead of building them.

A bit of organization would also help. Devise a weekly schedule. For example, you could do crunches without weights for the first half of the week and concentrate on weights in the latter part of the week.

And keep a wary eye on your diet. Do not eat fatty foods that build up fat faster than you can burn them through exercise.

Ab Gym Workouts – The 7 Habits Of Highly Effective Gym Goers

If you crave a firm and good looking abdomen, but can hardly keep pace with demanding ab gym workouts, this article is for you. So, go right ahead. Read about and emulate the 7 habits of highly effective gym goers, who:

1. Plan the Routine

Planning your workouts helps prevent interruptions that could easily divert you away from workouts. Prepare a routine and stick to it, no matter how strong the urge to skip and let go.

2. Use Resistance Training

Many believe strenuous workouts like aerobics or treadmill routines will get them the results they want. These do help reduce fat; however, building firm muscles calls for weight and resistance training. Ab gym workouts, involving resistance training, done properly and in accordance with a strict routine, will strengthen your abdominal muscles, and actually burn fat faster.

3. Select the Right Equipment

During ab gym workouts, start with low level weights and low resistance; your body is not tuned for strenuous workouts. Especially if you are a newbie, any sudden strain could tear your still weak muscles. A bench is easier to start with, as you get support for your back, and you do not have to bend more than 90 degrees, initially. Later on, you could graduate to weights and larger equipment, and then on, to an exercise ball that allows you to turn your body and train different sets of muscles at the waist.

Most importantly, learn to use gym equipment properly in your ab gym workouts. Faulty techniques can cause uneven muscle development, thereby marring your looks, instead of enhancing them.

4. Adopt the Right (Smart) Techniques

Space your ab gym workouts out, in intervals of short intense exercises involving different sets of muscles; repeat the cycle as many times as possible. Never ignore any signal from your body to stop. Increase the exercise intervals very gradually or you could endure muscle damage. Drink plenty of water; exercise can dehydrate your body and tire you out.

Workout buffs tend to overwork their muscles in their eagerness to train and develop muscles fast. Always stay within the limits of what your body can handle. During ab gym workouts, reserve some effort to train and strengthen your back muscles, as well. This could help prevent any unwanted injury as well as chronic back ache.

Choose a scientifically proven routine; avoid any unscientific antics gym colleagues might suggest.

5. Try Different Equipment Sets and Routines

Using the same routine every day — even if you are doing it diligently — will not give you the results you crave. There are different sets of abdomen muscles, and they all need to be strong, not only to make you look good but also to support your body properly. One set of strong muscles surrounded by another set of weak muscles will not improve matters in any way. Target all-round development.

6. Eat The Right Food

Overdosing yourself with oily and greasy stuff or fast food, even as you try your best to develop a muscular looking waist, will only waste your effort. Be a smart exerciser rather than a boring mechanical robot doing a routine without thinking about what you are doing or what you are aiming to achieve. Limit your food to a healthy and fiber rich diet including enough of the right kinds of fats. You also need those carbohydrates. And don't forget to drink plenty of water.

7. Rely On Progression Charts

Chart down the results of your ab gym workouts — regularly measure your waist line and your muscle tone. Do this for intervals of a week or more. The chart will reveal whether or not you are exercising correctly; you will also feel motivated when you see progress.

Ab Workouts for Women

Want a Great Ab Tone? Do Ab Exercises!

Do you wish your tummy was firm, not flabby, and that when you wear jeans, you didn't have abs that spilled over? Do you wish for flat abs so your significant other would always do a double-take whenever he sees your abs? You're not alone — most women wish those things and feel the way you do about flabby abs. These same women, however, believe that sexy flat abs is something they'd only get to have in their dreams. If you think a great ab is impossible for you to ever have, think again! You can have the ab of your dreams — but you need to work hard for it.

The first thing you need to do is stop thinking you can't ever get rid of all the extra fat on your belly. You can get started building your core muscles even if you've still got a lot of excess body fat. Just make sure that as you work on your midsection, you're also working on your whole body by doing cardiovascular exercises and following a healthy diet. The muscles you're building in your core and other parts are going to accelerate the fat burning process. Get your body so conditioned to working out that your muscles are going to be burning fat even if you're just sitting or sleeping.

To build those core muscles, you need resistance, and not just on your abdominal section. Contrary to what the infomercials will have you believe, you aren't going to develop a six-pack ab just by doing crunches all day. Also do some lunges, squats, and other weight resistance muscles. The muscles in your abs are too few and too little to burn all your extra body fat. You'll need to build your largest muscles instead.

Pilates is a good workout that a lot of women get into since its main focus is the core. Regardless of the Pilates exercise you're doing, you can be sure your core is being worked out so you can have the kind of ab you want.

To build muscles that will burn off the extra body fat, you need resistance training. However, you'll also want to do cardiovascular exercises to accelerate the calories that your muscles burn. You can walk, jog, run, or swim. Make sure you start out slow. Build up slowly — and all the while, don't forget your core. There are ab exercises you can do right now to build ab muscles even if you still have some flab hanging over it.

Start building your ab tone by doing leg crunches. Lie on the floor with your arms stretched out over your head. Slowly lift your legs to a 90-degree angle, contracting your abdomen in the process. Lower your legs back down just as slowly. Do as many leg crunches as you can without pain. Try to do leg crunches for 30 seconds.

There's another crunch you can do as you lie on the floor. Bend your knees at a 90-degree angle so that your lower legs are parallel to the ceiling. Then bring your knees toward your head and crunch your core. Do this exercise slowly and for about 30 seconds.

If you combine these two ab exercises with the other exercises you do, as well as stick to a good diet, it won't be long until you see those sexy flat abs.

Ab Exercises For The Ladies

Without a doubt, every woman would like to get rid of that unsightly flab around the abdominal area and have the leanest looking middle section. When you have a lean tummy you will feel more confident about yourself especially when wearing figure hugging outfits and bikinis.

That being said, in order to achieve this lean look, you will need to work for it; and as with everything else desirable in life it does not come easy. You will need to be dedicated to reaching your goals without getting impatient and frustrated. There are quite a number of ab workouts for women that if performed over a period of time will bring forth some very desirable results.

Sit-ups

One of the most common workouts for the middle section is the sit-up exercise. All you have to do is lie flat on the floor, preferably on an exercise mat; it would be better if you could have someone around to hold your legs down since your body will try to resist this workout. With the legs firmly held to the floor, place your hands behind your ears and lift your upper torso to an angle of 90 degrees; go back down and repeat the process.

With sit ups, try to do at least ten repetitions before resting after which you should start another set of the same number. Five sets of ten repetitions every day will work your ab muscles quite well; make sure that with each day you try to increase the number of repetitions per set.

Bicycle

Without a doubt, the bicycle workout is one of the most effective ab workouts for women. This workout will also involve lying on the floor; in this case, you will not need a helping hand. As the name suggests, the movements of the workout resemble those made when cycling. With your hands behind your head you will have to lift your right knee towards your chest; while holding that position, move your left elbow to meet the right knee. Once you have done that do the exact opposite. That is: bring your left knee to your chest and then move your right elbow meet it. For this work out to be more effective, you will need to perform these movements with speed.

Exercise Bar

Another very effective ab workout for the ladies involves the use of an exercise bar. First of all grab the bar with both hands such that your body is suspended from it, make sure that your feet are not touching the floor. You should then proceed to lift your legs until you make a 90 degree angle with your upper body; do a number of repetitions, rest and then do it all over again.

Swiss Ball

You can also use a Swiss ball to get a good ab workout. You will first need to get into the push-up position, now lift your legs and place them on top of the Swiss ball. Proceed on to sort of drag the ball with your feet making an acute angle between your calves and hamstring region and then straighten your legs; do so repetitively.

Ab Workouts for Firming

Most people who work out aim to have strong core sections. However, we're all formed a bit differently. This not only makes results variable for certain exercises, but it means that many workout machines just aren't built right for you. It is important to find workouts/exercises that will help you get firm abs.

One of the most neglected aspects of a firm core is workout variety. Most people end up doing the same sets of ab workouts over and over. As a result, they develop only a small set of muscles for only a few movements. Eventually, many of these muscles will peak and further development will be difficult, if even possible.

One of the nice things about working out your abdominal muscles is that you don't really need any equipment. Your body is built in such a way that you can do a variety of bodily movements in order to get full, firm abs. This is why workout routines, such as Pilates, have become so popular among those seeking tight cores. The variety of movements involved with Pilates that work out the core is so extensive that all of your core muscles can be worked out with an ever varying workout routine. Yet, Pilates tends to offer safe, fluid movements that people of any fitness level can do.

If you have a gym membership, you might as well be taking advantage of the machines at your gym that help you to do very safe ab workouts. Many of these machines can work out your abs in a variety of ways, but machines will never offer as much variety as free weights and free exercises. This is why it is great that most gyms have weight training instructors to assist you in setting up a workout plan to achieve your goals.

One of the popular tools incorporated into workouts by weight training instructors and that is inexpensive for use in the home is the exercise ball. The exercise ball allows you to target and work out wide muscle ranges in unique, yet natural motions. The fact that you must use some muscles to balance yourself on the ball while at the same time targeting a specific muscle set allows you to get a more complete workout.

Exercise balls are commonly used to target the abdominal muscles with a few specific exercises. The ab curl is very popular for this. Or, you can lie on your stomach across the ball and work out your oblique muscles, hip flexors, and rectus abdominus. Another popular ab firming routine involves lying on your back and putting the ball between your feet.

The key to doing workouts to get firm abs is to be consistent at getting abdominal exercise, but to do it in a variety of different ways. In other words, you need to have a plan for daily activity, but you don't have to do the same abdominal workouts each day. The more variety you get in your abdominal workouts, the more consistent and smooth the development of your abdominal muscles will be. So keep doing your workouts, but from a variety of different angles in order to give yourself the firm abs you desire.

Which Crunchless Ab Workouts Exercise is Best?

Most exercise buffs have abdominal muscles that are strong to a degree, albeit hidden behind a layer of fatty skin. Thanks to the fat, they just don't seem to be aware of it. They aspire for well toned abs, but shy away from doing "difficult" crunches. In this article, I take a look at the merits of various crunchless ab workouts that could prove the solution for people like you:

Reduced Food Intake:

Start by reducing fat intake in your food. This will cause your body to burn stored fat. But the human body first burns fat from parts other than the abdomen, so the results will be visible only after some time.

Jogging:

When jogging, try lifting your legs higher, so that your knees are level with your hip. Better still, try and lift them up to the level of your navel. You will soon see the results, as long as you do it consistently.

Toe Touching:

Without bending your knee, lift your leg up, straight. Now, try to touch your toes. Only use your ab muscles to help you reach your toes. This is not easy and you'll need flexibility. Warm up first, by jogging for a few minutes, always remembering to lift your knees high. If stiff muscles make it hard to keep your legs straight, try holding your toes and then straightening your legs. Lift your upper body a little while doing so.

Face Down Floor Exercise:

This is relatively difficult and you should only do it for a few seconds, at least initially. Lie face down on your exercise mat. Fold your feet inward, so that they rest on your toes. Now, keep your arms underneath your chest, elbows bent, and forearms pointed forward. Now, lift your body; hold this position, for a few seconds, or for as long as you can. Gradually, increase the duration you support yourself on the arm. Avoid bending your body downward during this workout. It needs lots of practice, and the results make it worth the while.

Lateral Floor Exercise:

Rest on one side of your body, and lift yourself using only your arm, bent at the elbow. Keep the rest of your body straight, and concentrate your entire weight on your elbow. Do not bend your body forward. Repeat this on the other side. This will strengthen the lateral and frontal muscles of your abdomen. Do this one only after warming up, or you could end up with a muscle sprain.

Twist:

This is among the crunchless ab workouts popular among athletes and soccer players. It involves standing side by side and passing a ball from one player to another. The twist motion strengthens the sides of the abdomen while straining the ab muscles also. The back benefits too, but take care not to overdo it.

Cycling Motion:

This is one of the crunchless ab workouts you can do lying down. Move your legs in a circular motion so as to simulate cycling. Instead of pointing your toes downward, parallel to your body, point them upward and keep them straight.

"Anywhere" Crunchless Ab Workouts:

You can do these, in almost any position, while sitting in a chair at your office or lying in bed at home. Pull your stomach simultaneously inward and backward towards the spine. Hold for a few seconds, and release. Repeat this process as many times as you can. This is akin to forcible exhalation of air or rapid breathing. You can alternate between pulling in the entire frontal abdominal muscle, or just the lower part. Relax for a few minutes and then you are ready to repeat.

Lower Ab Workout – Make the "Fab Four" Work for you

Lower ab workout routines are important because most of the fat collects in the lower abdomen. Stronger lower abdominal and back muscles also prevent lower back injury. In this article, I reveal 4 fab ways you can get your lower abs into shape, and the incidental additional hidden benefits you will get:

1. Legs' Crane

This is a simple yet most effective form of lower ab workout that is, at the same time, very strenuous. Lie flat on the floor, arms placed by your side, palms facing downward, beside your hips. Keep both legs together and stiff. Without bending your legs, lift them straight up to form a 45 degree angle with your body. Hold for three to four seconds or for as long as you can, and gradually lower your legs. Repeat 10 times; rest for a minute or two, and resume. Continue only as long as you are able to do this safely, without muscular injury. Stop if you feel any pain or are unable to continue.

Vary things a little and try to bring your legs together — as close to your upper body as possible. This will curl your lower back and strengthen your lower abdomen. The stretch you feel on the lower back will help relieve strain on your lower back. Do this only if you do not suffer any complications of the back. This workout is similar to a yoga posture and having a flexible body does help. Follow up this routine by exercising your back muscles and end with stretches. Do the complete set and you'll feel great.

2. Legs' Swirl

Though this lower ab workout is similar to the previous routine, once you've raised your legs to 45 degrees spread them a bit and swirl them. Move both legs – simultaneously – in opposite directions. Take care not to spread your legs too wide or you could end up spraining an inner-thigh muscle. This is not as easy as it may appear. To get the swirling motion right, imagine sitting by a swimming pool and dipping your legs in the water.

Vary this workout by spreading your legs simultaneously wide apart, and then bringing them together, thereby simulating a pair of scissors. Maintain your balance by keeping your arms a tad away from the body or you could experience pain in the lower abdomen and back.

3. Cycling Simulation

Lie flat on your back as though you were riding an imaginary bicycle. Raise your legs straight up, to 90 degrees, keeping your feet perpendicular to your legs. An extremely effective routine, this one benefits both your lower abdomen and lower back. Support your back by placing your arms by your side during this workout. Stop the moment you feel you can't go on.

4. Baby Curl

Lie flat on the floor with your arms by your side, palms pressed to the floor to support your body. Bring both legs together and lift them gradually, bent at the knees. Raise your chest gradually to bring your head towards the meeting point of your knees. Lock your arms around your legs and hold this position for a few seconds. Exhale slowly as you do this; similarly, inhale slowly, as you do the reverse. Lie flat and relax for four to five seconds. Repeat ten times.

Do this every morning. Begin with a warm up routine, and insure that there is little food in your stomach. To get the complete benefit from this routine, exercise your back, too. Lie flat, face down, and try to lift your upper body and your legs (kept close together) as you support yourself with your arms folded close beside you. This lower ab workout will strengthen your lower abdomen and back, alike, and thereby improve your posture.

Ab Workout Equipment — 4 Questions That Will Help Find The Best Gear

Getting six pack abs is not as easy as TV commercials would have you believe. You need to have steely determination, and know the right workout techniques. Most importantly, you'll need to use the best ab workout equipment. There is a range of equipment models to choose from, each with its manufacturer's tall claims. In this article, I discuss 4 questions to ask that will help insure you get the best equipment:

1. Is The Ab Workout Equipment Safe?

The first thing you should worry about is the safety of the equipment. Any gear that is clumsy, dangerous looking, and that requires you to bend through dangerous positions is hazardous. It could result in serious bodily harm. The equipment manuals should clearly describe the safest ways of using the equipment. If you find the positions difficult, or the manual does not give safety tips, then buying such equipment could result in serious injury that will take weeks to recover from. The injuries that can easily happen with the wrong type or use of ab workout equipment and which are most difficult to treat are injuries of the back, a muscle pull or strain of the abdomen, or a muscle tear. So, make safety your first concern.

2. How Much Are You Willing To Pay?

Most ab workout equipment is costly. Costly doesn't necessarily mean 'good'. How good the equipment is depends on how much it helps increase the intensity of your workouts. That alone would determine value for money.

3. Where Will You Keep The Equipment?

Almost all modern ab workout equipment sold on the market today appears compact. This is necessarily so, as homes are getting smaller and there is less space to store the equipment, let alone to exercise. So, look for equipment that fits snugly in your room, or probably in a corner, under a bed, or in a cupboard.

If you like to exercise as you travel, it would be a good option to buy compact equipment that you can carry with your baggage. This would help you maintain your exercise regimen even when you are away from home. Finding such compact exercise gear to suit your specific needs is not easy as you would not only have to consider the design, but you would also have to see how much it weighs.

4. Can You Adjust and Choose Between Different Levels Of Workout?

The ab workout equipment you choose should not restrict you to few workout positions. If that happens, it implies that you are not doing a proper workout. To do justice to your workout routine, you have to vary your position — your stride and length — and the amount of strain put on your muscles as you workout; the machine should have different levels of resistance. The equipment should not just help you strengthen your muscles but should also allow you to increase your stamina.

Simultaneously, the equipment must support your body properly. Being able to exercise comfortably without worrying is very important. Remember, no jerky movements, or you could either break the machine, or tear a muscle. If the exercise routine is tiresome and clumsy, you are likely to quickly give up exercising, altogether. The equipment you use should have a range of motion that allows you to use all your muscles in your mid section. That alone will insure a proper workout and you will notice a well developed waist. You get the well-toned look not only from burning fat but also from having a strong set of abdominal muscles.

6 Hot Reasons To Do Ab Roller Workouts

Many would love to have sexy flat abs like those flaunted by models on television. However, most of them simply cannot afford the expensive exercise equipment advertised on TV or simply don't have the time to exercise in a gym. If you are one of them, what do you do?

Stop worrying, for here comes help. You can depend on ab roller workouts to insure that you get those coveted trim and rock-hard abs. These workouts can make you look as good as the hotshot models on TV, and within a price and time-line you can certainly afford. Here are my 6 hot reasons why ab roller workouts are the best way to get sexy flat abs — or even six pack abs (depends on when you decide to cut back):

1. Concentrate On Abs
The pull ups that help strengthen your ab muscles require you to lift your upper body. A lot of energy is wasted in lifting just the head and chest while at the same time putting a lot of strain on your neck. The ab roller supports your head, neck and upper chest so that you are free to direct energy to the ab muscles which is really what you want to work on. Such support also reduces any chances of injury or strain of your neck and spine as the roller follows the natural curve of the spine.

2. Offer Variable Resistance Training
You can vary the level of difficulty or resistance of your exercise simply by moving your arms. Just holding the equipment at different positions during ab roller workouts can change the amount of pressure you apply during abdominal crunches. Once you have worked the front, you can concentrate on the sides and back. Changing positions during ab roller workouts could get you your best dividends.

3. Provide Quick Results
Adopt ab roller workouts, and you have the fastest way to develop your ab muscles. What's more, thanks to the unique posture of ab roller workouts, you are allowed to actually see your ab muscles being worked. You can adjust your position to concentrate on the

particular muscle you want to work with, thereby facilitating faster development of your ab muscles. No other type of workout provides such quick results.

4. Facilitate Safe Exercise

Even though there is hardly a way you will injure yourself with ab roller workouts, the guides provided with the rollers give enough instruction on safe use of the equipment. There are no weights surrounding you so you do not have to worry about injuring yourself through any accidents. You depend on the frame for ab roller workouts and do not have to use any resistance bands. This eliminates the chance of slippages and snapping of bands. The cage gives a feeling of safety as you only have to concentrate on workouts and nothing else.

5. Make It Easy For Newbies To Adapt

Beginners do not have to struggle to understand the equipment. Ab roller workouts can be done by a range of people, from newbies to professional body builders. During workouts, you simply have to concentrate on your belly, to make the muscles stronger.

6. Spare Your Wallet

Ab rollers are among the cheapest exercise equipment on the market that help tone your ab muscles. Expensive equipment doesn't necessarily mean great workouts and great abs. Ab roller workouts are as effective as they are inexpensive. As the equipment used employs a simple design you don't have to worry about spending a lot of money on equipment that will take up a lot of space. Ab roller workouts are arguably the cheapest way to build strong abs.

Can an Iron Gym Workout Be Effective?

An Iron-Gym workout depends on a simple looking bar or rod that attaches to a door frame and is a handy tool for upper body muscular development, using your own body weight for exercises. It is also among the cheapest forms of muscle building as you do not need to buy weights; instead, you lift yourself. All you need with this home gym equipment is the space between your door frames.

Can you really rely on an iron-gym ab workout to develop sexy flat abs? You certainly can, but not in any conventional way you might imagine. In this article, I explain exactly how it works.

The rod can hold up to 300 pounds and most people don't weigh that much. It's a high strength heavy duty steel rod weighing only six pounds with strong pads at the edges that fix to a door frame as you pull it down with your weight. These pads are especially designed to hold your weight, just make sure it's secured tightly to the frame.

The rod can be fixed to any door frame between 24 and 32 inches wide. To be able to grip and hold, the pads only need three and a half inches of width of door frame.

You will have to buy the "Ab Strap" that is sold as an accessory and used for the mid section and lower abdominal exercises. Once you have fixed the straps, you are ready to do your iron-gym ab workout.

Hang from the rod in mid air, bring your knees close together and lift them up to your chest. Bringing your knees close to your chest is not going to be easy, at least the first few times, and hence, you will need a lot of determination, apart from strength, to be able to do that. Once you have developed enough strength to achieve it, you can do 10 to 30 and up to 50 repetitions at a time, in order to strengthen your ab muscles. This set of exercises focuses on the lower section of the abdomen which is the part that usually protrudes in fat people.

You can also use the rod to exercise your abdomen by moving your legs through a cycling motion. Riding an imaginary cycle would not only strengthen your lower abdomen, but also help shape the upper part of your thighs, thereby ridding your hips of a flabby appearance. Hanging straight down from the rod, you can also try to lift your leg backwards. This requires strength and will gradually make your lower back strong, as you progress through your exercise regimen. However, you should be cautious, as an imperfect technique or angle can cause back ache, especially in weaker people.

Once you have managed to perfect the front lift technique, you can learn to swing your legs laterally as you lift them to strengthen the muscles on the sides of the abdomen. Again this is likely to be hard at first, but once you have enough strength, you will enjoy this swing motion as you lift your legs. Just remember to keep you knees together. At no point of the swing should you separate your knees. Doing this exercise with knees together prevents injuries like muscle sprain.

A useful variation of this process is to hang perpendicular to the rod and swing your legs sideways like a pendulum, while keeping your legs together. Just take care that nobody is coming through that doorway while you are doing this or you can cause a nasty accident, hurting yourself and others. You don't have to swing far, just a little to get the sides of your abdomen into the shape you desire.

Is An Exercise Ball Ab Workout Better?

An exercise ball ab workout offers some unique advantages you might not enjoy with other gym equipment. In this article I discuss some exercise routines you can do to develop trim abs using a simple exercise ball and analyze the advantages of this kind of workout.

Ball As Back Support:

You can do normal ab crunches by supporting yourself on the ball. Exercise ball ab workout crunches are done with your lower back supported on the ball. Do not sit on the ball and lean back or you could roll over – providing amusement to everybody else in the gym. Relax on the ball, as if you were sitting on a high-cushioned sofa; lean back, with your arms locked behind your neck. Bend forward, as in a normal ab crunch, and repeat this routine, eight to twelve times. Rest, and repeat. Initially, you might struggle to maintain your balance and simultaneously engage the muscles in your leg, hip and back along with the abdomen.

Ball As Support For Feet:

Lie down on the floor, with your feet placed on the ball, for support. Pull up your upper body as far as you can, using the abdominal muscle. If it's hard to keep your legs together on the ball, try crossing your legs to lock them in place. Try not to let your legs roll off the ball. Keeping your eyes fixed to your knees as you pull yourself up will help center your head, at the knees. This should help prevent any sprain in your neck and back.

Chair & Ball:

An exercise ball ab workout variation involves using a chair. Use a smaller ball; lie down on the floor facing the chair with your legs slightly apart, kept on the chair. Place the ball over your groin and start rolling it upward till you reach your knee and beyond. Gradually roll back the ball, to the groin. You should do this particular routine slowly. Any jerky movement or carelessness on your part could cause you pain in the lower abdomen. Breathe slowly, exhaling as you rise and inhaling as you go back to your prone position.

Knee High Ball:

You'd need powerful arms for this one. Choose a ball which is up to your knee in height. Get down on all fours, facing away from the ball. With your arms stiffened, as in a push-up stance, raise both your legs onto the ball and keep your back straight to form a straight line. Hold this position for as long as you can. Lower one leg at a time to rest, and repeat. This is a great way to strengthen your mid section which is normally known as the core of the body.

So, what unique advantages does this type of workout give you?

To start with, the exercise ball allows you to balance your body by engaging different muscles and not just one particular muscle which is not possible with any other equipment. This improves both your coordination and your reflexes. Also, this ab routine is accepted by experts as an important part of programs for weight loss.

Apart from the range of exercises you can do with the exercise ball, you can also easily change positions – by sliding over the ball, or rolling the ball, along the floor. If necessary, you could roll it on a wall to exercise your legs, back and front.

All in all, the ball is an inexpensive yet very useful piece of equipment. Use it in the gym or at home according to your convenience.

Can Couch Potatoes Get Six-Packs Doing Chair Ab Workouts?

Yes, we can! It is actually possible to sit in a chair and work out to get fab abs. In this article, I explain exactly how you can use chair ab workouts to get trim abs.

The chair that you'd normally use in a gym is called the Captain's Chair. You don't actually sit in this chair. You stand straight, supporting your back, mid section and lower back against the padding provided on the chair. Place your arms firmly and rigidly on the armrests to support your bodyweight. Once you have secure support on the extended armrests, bring your knees close together and try to lift your legs up and close to your chest. Do not bend your back. With any swinging motion, you are liable to injure your back as you bang against the pads. Likewise, don't swing your legs sideways or you will hurt yourself.

You might find this a bit hard in the beginning; hence, you can start with lifting your leg up to your hip. You will see gradual improvement. You can do about 12 repetitions at a time then stop; rest for a few seconds, and repeat the whole process again. Once you are sure you can handle closed knee lifts, you can try variations like a cycling motion or lifting your legs while keeping them straight, always remembering not to bend them at the knee. When you lift your legs — without bending them — be sure to support your lower back well, against the chair, or you could hurt yourself. This workout is best done under the guidance of a gym instructor.

There are other types of chair ab workouts that you can try in a seated position. The equipments used for this purpose are chairs that either do or do not support your back. These have tension bands for resistance, and function similar to ab crunches, except that you have to do these crunches seated on a chair instead of lying on a mat on your back.

Some workout chairs come equipped with back rests, thereby allowing you to rest your back as you pull your entire upper body forward while the knee support helps hold your legs in position. Most of these chairs have two resistance bands, usually one each at the front and back. You'll find these much better to use than chairs that do not have a support for the back.

In respect of chairs, which are not equipped with back supports, you would need to grip the extended tension bands — usually on the sides — and pull your entire upper body forward in order to try and touch your knee with your forehead. Most such chairs will have a pair, or more, of tension bands. You can choose to use additional bands, according to your individual strength. Take care not to lean back or you could topple over and hurt yourself. As you continue with your workout regimen with these chair ab workouts, you will gradually feel your ab muscles hardening.

A major advantage of chair ab workouts is that you do not have to strain your back and neck, as you well might when you do conventional abdominal crunches. Since you do not have to grip your neck or head, it helps prevents back injury and any unnecessary strain on your neck. You can be free from the worry of backache, and you also focus much of your energy on your ab muscles than you normally would when raising your upper body up from floor level. This is an additional benefit you get with ab chair workouts that is conspicuously absent with conventional ab crunches done on the floor.

Is An Ab Workout Program All "Just Hype"?

Virtually everywhere you look for weight loss information, you are likely to find an ab workout program, ostensibly devised "just for you". In this article, I help you cut through the clutter, and find out if it makes sense. First, define the problem:

Information Illusion:

Too much information about any ab workout program, delivered in a short time, is liable to confuse you, thereby impairing your judgment. Go beyond information overload and judge the benefits, if any, to you — as an individual.

Tall Temptation:

TV ads that feature attractively built models always promise results in a few days. But you probably know you cannot lose weight and strengthen muscles by relying on either exercise or diet, alone. If TV models told the truth, they would admit that their trim abs have resulted from hours of toil, combined with a planned diet.

"Guaranteed" Gimmick:

TV ads that promise quick results back up their claims with strong irresistible "money back" guarantees. You might be tempted to try it as you are apparently not losing anything. But you could get so frustrated and distrusting that you might end up skipping a genuine ab workout program suited to you.

So, is it all just hype? Not if you know how to get past the sales spiel to the real solution lurking behind.

Time Trap:

Many either have lots of time for exercise, or can barely manage an hour a day. Your ab workout program should allow you to repeat a set of exercises, daily, and also give you some time for rest. If you are rushing off to work or tend to get busy with household chores, without a break, you are denying your body rest, which, in turn, is liable to cause serious injury.

A different series of ab crunches planned and done daily over a week, with rest on Sundays, will work much better than spending many hours for a day or two and doing nothing for the next few days.

If you are a gym goer and there are many people waiting for the same equipment, plan your routine and share it with your gym mates, so as to avoid conflict.

Motivation Maze:

If you tend to start with a big bang and then peter out in a couple of months, like your new year's resolutions, you probably have already wasted a lot of time and energy.

Choose an ab workout program that does not tire you easily, one that you enjoy and can stick with. Select an easy set, like jogging for a few minutes followed by a few minutes of stretching, some crunches of the front and sides, a few of the back (necessary to prevent back injury), and a few pushups or chin ups. Then, stretch or slow jog again to relax your muscles, and rest, finally. A wholesome exercise routine should make you feel energetic while your abdominal muscles feel stronger by the day.

If you exercise in a gym, schedule your routine with the help of an instructor, to avoid competing with others. Choose the equipment carefully and adjust the weights or resistance in keeping with your stamina level.

Diet Decoy:

Consuming a low calorie diet during an exercise cycle trims body fat and builds strong muscles. Incorporate this into your plan and you won't have to worry about an extra helping of cake or bite of ice-cream. No harm in treating yourself once in a while.

Equipment Enticement:

You don't have to depend on expensive equipment you see in gyms. Only use equipment that increases your intensity of exercise over a period, while not costing you much. Your equipment should allow you to graduate to a higher level from that of the beginner.

Ab Workout Routine Mistakes

Most people would prefer to either have six-pack abs or flat abs. But desiring something and having the discipline to learn how to do your ab workout the right way on a regular basis are two different things. You have little chance of success if you don't set up a good ab workout routine and stick to it.

A common mistake is a failure to increase workout intensity. At the same time, you need to increase workout intensity slowly. The difficulty is in determining just how hard you should push yourself. You need to work out the muscles, but you don't want to strain them.

You can think of your ab workout routine the same way you think of taking a walk for exercise. Walking isn't something that exhausts you, but we know from studies that it does improve health if it is done consistently over time. The catch is that you must increase your pace and distance up to a reasonable amount over the course of your first few years in order to continue to increase your cardiovascular health. You don't have to put yourself at risk of injury to stay in good health in this way, just as you don't have to violently attack your ab muscles to improve their strength.

Of course, the greatest mistake you can make when working out is working out incorrectly. This is just as true with ab workouts as any other workouts. Your exercises need to target your abdominal muscles using natural movements. You have to be particularly careful that you are actually working out your abdominal muscles. Many people compensate for resistance difficulties by using their leg or back muscles. This can of course cause injury, and does nothing to improve abdominal tone.

You need to learn how to recognize where you're feeling the tension when you work out so as to be certain that you're working out the proper regions. With your ab workout routine, you can help this process along by tightening your ab muscles for your workouts just as if someone is about to deliver a blow to your gut.

It is generally a good idea to avoid any workout routines that require you to bend over and round your back against hard objects or bear heavy weights. Back injuries are common when weight training is done improperly. If you remember the old style of doing crunches by pulling your neck forward to your knees, you can understand why so many back injuries occurred. You don't have to injure yourself to get a good ab workout. Don't bother with risky ab workout routines, as injuries will only set you back.

Avoiding ab workout routine mistakes is a key to successfully developing toned abs, whether you want six pack abs or flat abs. You can take things a step further by experimenting with interval workouts, which can also benefit your overall health. Make sure you eat right and get plenty of cardiovascular exercise. A complete lifestyle and a disciplined study of ab workout basics will ensure that you get the best possible results.

#

EXCERPT from *Ab Workouts for Hardgainers*

Building Muscle without Weights

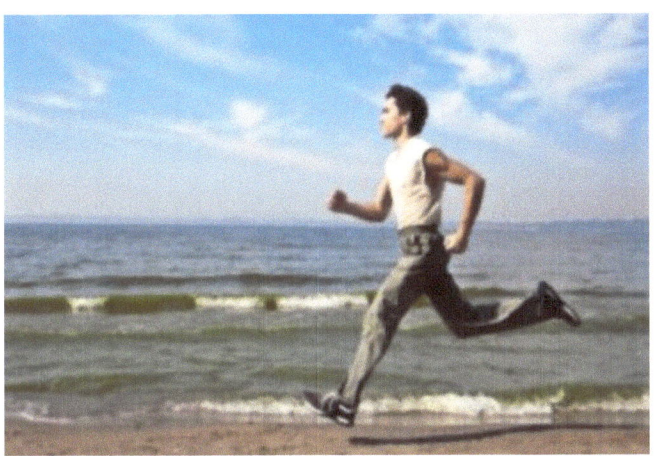

There are dozens of effective ways to build muscle mass without weights. Sometimes it's even more efficient. It's certainly more convenient — no trips to the gym — and can be safer, too. It's not an either/or proposition, either. You can do both and get the unique benefits of each body building approach.

Consider the simple, traditional push-up. Do them the traditional way and you'll get some cardio benefit and help build your biceps, triceps, and back muscles (lats) to a certain degree. But to really increase their size and clearly define them you need weights, right?

Not necessarily. Anything that makes the muscles involved in push-ups work harder will necessarily stimulate blood flow and the growth of muscle proteins in the body. Here are just a few ways to do that.

Change the angle of your body. Instead of lying with your feet on the floor, put them on a chair, a footstool, the couch, the steps of your deck… anywhere safe and stable. Gravity then requires you to exert extra force to raise your torso by the same amount you would normally. Simple, no?

The results will speak for themselves. You'll get well-defined biceps and bigger pecs if you stick to a regular routine. You can work your way up, and make it even tougher, by gradually increasing that angle. Then, for a variation, try those same push-ups with only one arm at a time.

The same technique can be used to enhance the effectiveness of sit-ups. Ordinary sit-ups help burn calories, as well as define and strengthen your abdominals, glutes, and lats. Working those large muscles (not the only ones that get a workout, of course) helps you achieve that great look you want to impress the ladies and feel good. Work them harder and get more of those muscle-mass building and weight loss benefits. Here's how…

Instead of doing the classic "lie flat on your back on a level surface with your toes under the couch, put your hands behind your head…," vary the method.

One helpful variation is simply, again, to change the angle. Select a comfortable, smooth surface that's at an angle. That could be an incline board. Or, you could seek out a slanted sidewalk and use a mat. Find a smooth stretch of grass on a hill. Then do your normal number of reps and sets.

End of Excerpt – but not the end of this chapter.

For more information on *Ab Workouts for Hardgainers*, check out its page on Amazon.com or Google Books.

DISCLAIMER

Information presented here is for educational purposes only.

Your use of these materials for anything other than educational purposes is STRICTLY AND TOTALLY YOUR RESPONSIBILITY. YOUR USE OF ANY OF THIS INFORMATION CONSTITUTES YOUR ACCEPTANCE OF YOUR PERSONAL RESPONSIBILITY FOR ANY POSSIBLE CONSEQUENCES OF SUCH USE.

EXERCISES NOT PERFORMED WITH PROPER TECHNIQUE COULD CAUSE PERSONAL INJURY.

WE DISCLAIM ANY RESPONSIBILITY FOR YOUR USE OF THIS INFORMATION.

IF YOU DO NOT ACCEPT RESPONSIBILITY FOR YOUR OWN ACTIONS, DO NOT USE THIS INFORMATION!

Recommended Books

Ab Workouts for Hardgainers ---- by Michael Weston
Basic Ab Workouts Give You Sexy Flat Abs – Michael Weston

Digital Books by Joyce Zborower

Click here to go to my Amazon page

-- MYSTERIES/SHORT STORIES

The Trust – a cautionary tale
Little Mysteries – a short story

-- CRAFTS BOOKS

Handcrafted Jewelry Step by Step – 6 intermediate and advanced original designs
Handcrafted Jewelry Photo Gallery – cast jewelry -- fabricated jewelry
Wire Jewelry Photo Gallery – Original Designs
Creations in Wood Photo Gallery – jewelry boxes, screens, storage ideas
Bargello Quilts Photo Gallery – quilt wall hangings
Bargello Train Quilt – cutting and sewing instructions
Sell Your Work – how to turn your craft into your business

-- FOOD/NUTRITION RELATED BOOKS

No Work Vegetable Gardening – for in-ground, raised, or container gardening
How to Eat Healthy – foods to eat . . . foods to avoid
The Truth About Olive Oil – benefits, curing methods, remedies
External Uses of Extra Virgin Olive Oil – Folk Remedies ... Body Lotions ... Pet Treatments
Signs of Vitamin B12 Deficiencies – Who's at Risk – Why – What Can Be Done
13 Easy Tomato Recipes – nature's lycopene rich superfood for heart health and cancer protection
3 Fruit Pie Recipes – apple, cherry, crisp persimmon

BBQ Spare Ribs Recipe – with homemade honey BBQ sauce

-- *PSYCHOLOGY BOOKS*

Different Types of Depression – Characteristics and Treatments

Psychology of Success – how to have success when trying to change how you look

How to Fight Depression – 9 case studies ---- by John F. Walsh

Emergency Services Mental Health Professional – Memoirs and Experiences – John F. Walsh

-- **CHILDREN'S BOOKS**

Christmas ABCs – cute animal illustrations

Baby Pics Counting and Number Book -- 1-13 The numbers are in numerals and words with lots of photos of babies.

Most of the above are also available as print-on-demand paperback editions. Also:

Grandma's No Work Vegetable Gardening – (paperback edition) same as *No Work Vegetable Gardening* except the photos are B&W and the price is lower.

Español Libros (Spanish language Books) – Available or Coming Soon

Haga click aquí para ir a mi página de Amazon --

http://amzn.to/MlKKpJ

El Fideicomiso – fábula con moraleja

Pequeños Misterios– cuento

Joyas Hechas a Mano Paso a Paso – diseños originales para nivel principiantes e intermedio

Joyas Artesanales Galeria de fotos – Joyas fundidas – joyas forjadas

Joyas de Alambre - Galería de fotos – Diseños originales

Creaciones en Madera- Galería de fotos – joyeros, biombos, ideas de almacenaje

Quilts Estilo Bargello - Galería de fotos – tapices de quilt

Quilt Tren en Bargello– instrucciones para cortar y coser

Vende tuTrabajo – como transformar tu arte en negocio

Signos de deficiencia de vitamina B12 -- Quén esta en riesgo – Por qué – Qué puede hacerse

La Psicología del Éxito – cómo tener éxito al tratar de cambiar tu apariencia

Huerto sin Esfuerzo – para jardinería en el suelo, elevada o en contenedor

Como Comer Sano – comidas para comer…comidas para evitar

La Verdad Acerca del Aceite de Oliva– beneficios, métodos de curación, remedios

3 Recetas de Pie de Fruta -- Manzana, Cereza, Caqui fresco

13 Recetas de Tomate Fáciles -- Superalimentos de la naturaleza ricos en licopeno para la salud del corazón y protección contra el cáncer

Receta de Chuletas de Cerdo en Barbacoa -- con salsa casera de barbacoa con miel

Fotos de Bebés Libro de Números y de Contar De 2 a 5 años – 1 - 13

ABCs de Navidad – Para niños de 2 a 5 años

Italian Language Books

La verita su olio de oliva **...** Prestazoini – Metodi di polimerizzazione -- Rimidi

Other Recommended Books

The Confession of a Trust Magnate ----- by George Allen Yuille

Picture the combined navies of the world anchored off our seaboard cities, the combined armies of the world in possession of our inland cities, envoys from each nation congregated at Washington partitioning our country, the entire population being apportioned as slaves to do the bidding of the conquerors.

Would you be interested?

*An equally appalling situation confronts
the people of this country to-day.
Read of it in the pages of this book.*

This book was written in 1911. Its message is critical for today – 2013.

One Last Thing Before You Go. . .

Thank you for purchasing ***Basic Ab Exercises Give You Sexy Flat Abs.***. If you enjoyed it, would you take a few minutes and write a short testimonial on its Amazon page? Your opinion is important to me and I do read all messages and use your ideas to help improve work going forward.

Also, please let your friends who also enjoy olive oil know about it on Facebook and Twitter? They will thank you. . . as will I.

Best ever,
Michael Weston